JAKE

Our Family's Encounter

with

TRAUMATIC BRAIN INJURY

Marion McCann

"Jake got hurt bad last night."

Carroll Gant Biggs-November 6th, 1995.

JAKE GOT HURT BAD LAST NIGHT

Our daughter's wedding had been as beautiful as any I have ever seen at Trinity United Methodist Church in Ruston, Louisiana. As a mother, I could not have been more pleased for her that evening as I witnessed the unfolding pages of her "storybook" wedding to her prince charming. It was what they call, a nice affair.

All the preparations, which I couldn't attend to, due to my traveling job, were taken care of with the help of close friends who helped her plan the evening from the invitations right down to picking out her wedding dress and dresses for all her lovely bridesmaids, even a cute little tux for Tyler her two year old son who was to serve as ring bearer...but, sadly, even now I am not sure if he was allowed the privilege since I only recall the wedding advisor for the church telling me,

"I don't like surprises."

She was uneasy about him being so young.....and; now, to verify if he did or did not, I would have to look back over photos from the wedding. I can't force myself to do it. A part of me wishes I could simply forget everything that happened the night of November 5, 1995. In my very worst nightmare, I never could have dreamed that our family would go from being so happy only to endure a horrendous, life-altering event in one night. An event so severe that it would adversely affect each one of us throughout all the days of our lives.

As the lovely wedding ceremony was ended and all the pictures were taken, we moved the wedding party to the Holiday Inn for the reception. Afterwards, my last duty for the week, as mother of the bride, was to drive the newlyweds to the Dallas-Fort Worth International Airport for their early morning flight to Mexico.

For my own safety's sake getting home, I picked up Cousin Dee in Shreveport to drive, while I napped from the airport, back to her home in Shreveport. (I planned to head for the car and get in the passenger's seat as soon as the plane took off with the kids for their honeymoon trip.) This sleep deficit I keep harping on, the part it played, was due to many miles on the highway as a long-distance trucker and the rest of the work week arranging for the caterer, lining up a bar maid and security to make sure no underage drinking got by us...renting and decorating a large conference room at the local Holiday Inn and almost forgetting to pick up the tickets to Cancun from the travel agency!

On Thursday night, I spent extra hours making sure the house and patio were in perfect order to have a memorable outdoor rehearsal dinner. We were meeting the grandparents of the groom for the first time on Friday evening and I wanted everything to be a good reflection of our family. Whatever extra effort it took in giving a warm welcome was important to me even if the cost would be more of my precious sleep.

I can remember telling everyone that I liked adding to my world, not taking away! (Yeah, I know. Who doesn't?)

Here is where "tired" figures in, on the drive over to the airport, my mind drifted back to yesterday's unsettling event of the morning in the choir room. I was contentedly ironing my daughter's wedding dress...an odd thing occurred. The area of the satin dress draped across the ironing board became as a TV screen....and on this screen, for an instant in time, I could see our oldest boy, his eyes closed, lying in a hospital bed with tubes and wires connected to him. I blinked and looked a second time then looked up at the clock in the choir room....it showed the time to be 11:30. I looked back at the dress and the image was gone.

After a few moments passed, my husband called to tell me that everything was okay but we had just heard from a deputy. He was letting us know that our son had run off the road and across his lawn making deep ruts. (It just happened to be the same deputy who was to work our security that night.) He was not going to ticket him and was glad he was not hurt but wanted us to know about the incident. I told John I hoped he told the deputy we would make sure our son fixed those ruts! How embarrassing but I knew it could have been far worse.

When I am overly tired, weird things happen such as this "vision thing" which I didn't share with anyone since it had resolved nearly as quickly as it had manifested itself.

As a long-distance truck driver, I've had my share of "dreaming with my eyes open" and on those occasions know it is past the time to pull over! However, this image on the dress had seemed more of a premonition than a dream...and, the phone call from John had proven to me it was indeed a premonition...but, now, the worst was over; my son was safe. I felt could relax and proceed with all the activities and festivities ahead.

I had been forewarned and now I should be fine since he was actually alright. (My thought on this is that the Holy Spirit allows me these times of strange occurrences because all of Heaven knows that I have such a hard time accepting loss.)

Maintaining control is the name of the game in the work I do, hauling hazardous chemicals in a tanker all across the nation. (Not that it matters now, but at that time, I was hauling nitro-glycerin in suspension from a plant in nearby Sterlington; although this was the safest way for it to be transported, I felt a degree of great responsibility to be an ultra-cautious driver.) Distractions can prove fatal.

My belief is that I am allowed a small grace of premonitions to warn me when bad times are coming so I can brace myself and make good decisions, even in the worst of times.

When you get behind the wheel of any vehicle, you need to be able to leave all your problems behind and pay full attention to safe driving. (Not to come off as a complete weirdo or a religious fanatic, but in years past, I have made believers out of the family when I announced an impending death within one day of our losses of family members.) I don't think I am special. I do think we all have potential to be a tad psychic when necessary ...and it is all the work of the Lord!

Anyhow, back to the story: It was 279 miles to DFW from the Holiday Inn at Ruston, Louisiana....we finally got there and the kids went inside to check their baggage and whatever else that had to be done before boarding the 6:15AM flight.

I got parked and walked into the terminal. I found a central spot to sit for the wait. Those fabric-covered, metal chairs that are bolted together looked uncomfortable enough to prevent a nap and they were just what I needed.

I reached for a discarded a newspaper, I have never forgotten the awful stories on the front page. A young mother had run her car off into a pond in the Carolinas and drowned her two little boys....on purpose. O.J. Simpson had also made the news. My eyes were locked on his picture but I wasn't seeing him. I was unable to get the horror off my mind of what the poor little boys' last moments must have been. I was also thinking how some women would give anything in this world to have just one child and here this lunatic was, murdering hers...a few minutes later, I heard my name on a loudspeaker.

It was a message that went something like this: "Marion McCann, please go to the nearest phone. You have a call on line four."

It was my Daddy! (Oh! How just like him to call; he was always so considerate.) He asked if the little couple had boarded...I happily told him, "No, but they just saw their luggage going up the loading ramp. They are close to taking off!"

I felt at ease and truly comforted to hear from Daddy after the busy couple of days and the tiring drive last night....yes, it was just like him to check on how things were going with us.

He never could have prepared me for his next words. I know if he could have done so, he would have handled everything different. His sentence left me stunned, "Jake got hurt bad last night."

I felt my heart freeze in my chest then my words came, "Is he going to make it?"

"We don't know yet. Do you want to ask Elisabeth and Jeff if they want to go on to Cancun under these circumstances? Let them know Jake would want them to do so."

Waving frantically to get their attention; I shouted as they approached, ""Jake got hurt bad last night. He would want y'all to go on your honeymoon."

They looked at each other and said in unison, "Honeymoon's over!"

I asked Daddy, "Is he at Lincoln General?"

"No. LSU-Med, ICU. We're all here. John followed the ambulance. Let Dee or Jeff drive if you need to. Y'all be careful. I'll be watching for you."

Jeff went to get their luggage back. My cousin and Elisabeth followed me to find the car. We were quiet. I guess we were in shock....Jeff finally came with the luggage. We got on I-20, eastbound before a word more was spoken.

"Mama? What happened?"

"Don't know. Forgot to ask. Just pray he lives through it."

Elisabeth began to cry. Cousin Dee began to pray aloud and that seemed to soothe Elisabeth.

The drive to LSU-Med was 200 miles from DFW....the only talking we did was when Dee or Jeff would ask if they could drive and I would refuse. I knew if I was not busy doing something, I'd begin to think and I didn't want to think. Thinking would change nothing. Crying would change nothing. I suppose the others were just like me, sending up one prayer after another. Praying that God would help Jake hang on. Praying that it would not be real bad....but in our hearts, we knew the truth. Daddy would not have called if he knew for certain Jake would pull through.

Back to the story: We made it to the big hospital in Shreveport...glad I had my cousin with me for directions; I had no idea where it was.

So many steps to climb...it seemed to take forever to make it up all the steps and through the main lobby, to an elevator...the elevator hummed its mechanical tune. It stuck in my head for the next month or longer....anytime I was not thinking, I could hear the distinct hum of that elevator.

(I'm old enough now to know it was probably my blood pressure..)

Finally reaching the floor, we stepped out and Daddy was standing right there, ready to show us to the ICU Waiting Room. We met up with John and many others who were already assembled there.

(A friend asked me recently what happened when I got to the floor where Jake was in ICU. I wish I could say that when I stepped from the elevator, I ran to my father's arms for consolation. I have tried to dredge up how it was when I entered the ICU Waiting Room, how my husband's composure was in those first moments of our realized tragedy: was he glad to see me? What did he say to me? Did he console our daughter? The answers are: I am not sure...truth is, I don't recall a thing of that nature. I know me and I know I was totally focused on absorbing all I was being told in case I needed to make a decision. There is no other memory to share.)

John told me how it happened. Jake had gotten a ride home with his best friend and they never made it to the house. The truck hit the tree at the top of our driveway, on the passenger side...hit so hard that the door popped open and even though Jake was wearing a seatbelt, his head got lodged in the opening between the frame of the truck and the door against the tree. No telling how long they had been trapped in the truck. The wrecker got there but had no chain to pull the truck away from the tree and had to go back to get one. Crucial minutes lost and more would be lost as one obstacle after another cropped up.

The ambulance arrived. The ambulance attendant slashed Jake's arm using his own pocket knife to cut the seatbelt. This was the least of his injuries.

The trip to our local hospital was the next of many more delays; and, get this: an orderly in the ER would not give John a blanket for Jake! Told him, it was no use. Jake was gonna die. (John got one himself out of the blanket warmer cabinet. If his boy died, he was gonna die in a warm blanket!)

Then the decision to air-lift was a failure...they got Jake loaded in the chopper but it wouldn't start. So, they moved him back in the ambulance and took off for LSU-Med with John following in his truck ...and then, as luck would have it, the ambulance got into the only traffic jam I have ever heard of Ruston having--before or since. (There was some kind of street dance or possibly just the crowd spilling out onto Hwy 80 at a place called Muther's.)

John was behind the ambulance and although he tried to navigate around the crowd, he got detained. (We have never understood why the ambulance driver did not head straight up 167 North to I-20 and save critical minutes.)

All these years later, I try to visualize John driving his pick-up truck and looking ahead for the ambulance carrying our precious cargo to the Shreveport hospital...would he have thought to put on his flashers? Was he clenching his teeth as I was on my drive from DFW? Was he driving 90 miles an hour like he did when our baby, Gabriel, was turning blue and we thought he would die before we got to the ER at St. Francis in Monroe? I can only wonder. I never asked and I don't really want to know...but that had to be the longest 80 mile trip he has ever driven.

The ambulance had reached LSU-Medical Hospital before him and the first person he met at the door to ER had been waiting for him...wanting to talk to him about organ donation.

Someone told me that either a priest or a minister or both had also come to greet him. I cannot imagine how John kept his composure and didn't collapse with a heart attack after getting that kind of reception. (It took dummy-me several years to realize that it was all about harvesting Jake's organs...not to get him any replacements. Jake was at death's door and everyone thought so but me. What was I thinking...so full of hope, I couldn't see the negatives.

Thank you, Jesus. You sustained me with hope and courage as no other could.)

It was not long after we sat down when the nurse came to the waiting room door and said to follow her. We could go in and see Jake.

A note to my reader: It is difficult emotionally for me to write this but I want you to know what happened with our family's first encounter of Traumatic Brain Injury. I might have something of value to say. When Jake was hurt, I would have been thankful to have had information about what people went through but there was nothing to be found.

For years, people have encouraged me to share the story of our tragedy so others in similar circumstances may be able to find some answers, some help, some hope and encouragement. I wanted to do this but the time never seemed to be right. When the time did seem right, no words would flow. If I so much as caught myself thinking back to that time, I immediately tried to focus on any and everything else. It is not a good memory.

I can remember the content of my prayers both the ones spoken out loud and also said repetitiously in my mind. They went mostly like: Please, Lord, let him live. Please let us keep him a little longer...I know he's yours…. but you loaned him to me and I'm not ready to give him back. I've only had him 18 years…wherever I've failed him as a mother, I'll make up for it. I promise You, I'll do better for him than ever before, if you please let me keep him…just a little longer, Lord.

I was always taught we should never try to bargain or make deals with God. I think it is important to tell you that I did it anyway….every chance I got.

In rehashing that time so many years ago, some parts are freshly recalled and some are painfully surfacing for the first time. For instance: I just thought of some of the last private times I had with my son. One was just before the wedding ceremony began. He had gotten dressed in his tux in one of the Sunday School rooms; he called down the hall for me. "Mom, you gotta come see this! These clothes really fit me and I feel good in them. I'm gonna dress like this all the time when I grow up. Do I look okay?"

"Yes! You do!" I know I had on a big happy smile.

He smiled at himself in the mirror.

[We proudly kept a picture on display at the hospital for all to see and in the nursing home.   It is a picture from that night, probably 3 hours before the wreck. It is of him and his two brothers and their father,

John, all so handsome and dressed so nicely. (I am glad we have that one picture of my four men all together for the last time.) Jake is extra handsome in that photo because not only was he a nice looking young man but also he was so proud of how he appeared in his rented tuxedo.]

Bear with me: after all these years, I am just now remembering the last conversation I had with Jake that night! We were at the Holiday Inn after the wedding reception: we left John in charge of little Tyler and the last minute duties, the good-byes and thanks to the guests and went outside together. We got in his truck....he gave me a ride to the house where I changed clothes in my 18-wheeler because that is where my main stash of comfortable clothes were kept...he pulled the old white Cadillac around to the truck for me.

I got in the car, ready to leave and said, "Be careful, Jake."

"I will, Mom. You, too! Love you."

Those were his last words to me as I left to pick up the newlyweds.

The ICU

I always heard the term "being on somebody's heels." We were a short few steps behind the nurse! It was Sunday morning, November 6th 1995. She led us through the double-swinging, stainless steel doors marked ICU and about 3 beds down on our left, we were stopped. To my utter horror, I was looking at the same image on Elisabeth's gown from yesterday. Our Jake was so hurt that his face was swollen out of proportion. At first glance, he didn't look like Jake. He looked like his big brother on the wedding gown!

I said, "This is not Jake!" Everyone looked sadly in my direction probably thinking all mother's deny the obvious at a time like this. I took a deep breath and raised my eyes to the clock. My blood literally ran cold. I was staring at the same type clock in the choir room...the same time, 11:30.

My whole world immediately shrank to the perimeter of this hospital bed. Jake was in some kind of constant motion; continually moving both his arms with clenched fists as if he were lifting weights....down by his sides then up to chest level....again and again and over again. I wanted that stopped!

John said, "We are told not to try to stop his arms from doing that."

The pain I felt standing there helpless to stop the terrible motions is indescribable. This pitiful scene of his hands gripped around an imaginary bar and arms jerking up from the mattress, teen-age muscles bulging with the work effort to chest level; then relaxing back to his sides only a moment before they jerked the unseen weights and bulged all over again...and again. Gut wrenching to watch.

I wanted to scream but clenched my jaws and watched the exertion Jake was involuntarily making instead. I said, "John, I don't care what they say, let's help him stop that." I was feeling light-headed. I knew Jake was expending precious energy and burning calories that could not be replenished if he remained in a state not able to eat.

"There is no way we can stop him. It's a reflex. It's called 'posturing' and it happens sometimes with bad head-injuries."

I felt my chest growing tight and I thought I was about to be sick or faint. I braced myself on the guard rail beside Jake as he continued to perform his futile task. I looked at John. He told me that Jake had been posturing all night long from the time John found him pinned in the truck against the tree. I never will forget how it felt seeing our child so hurt that his Mama's kisses couldn't make it better and all his Daddy's skills couldn't fix it this time.

I was wondering how long can anyone keep this physical action up and not bring on a heart attack? So many thoughts were chasing themselves around in my mind and none of them made sense.

I said nothing….just stared at the hole in the base of Jake's throat and a big flexible clear plastic tube running across to a machine. The sound of whirring was another affront to my sensibilities and a wave of nausea washed over again.

"They had to give him a tracheotomy. This is a 'trach' tube; he is being helped to breathe. That equipment is called a ventilator. The air sent in is regulated in volume and a certain pace and in temperature. It's breathing for him. He's on life-support."

John patiently explained what each wire was hooked up to ...and why it was where it was ...and what it was doing there. He showed me all the monitors and pointed out the thing that was implanted in Jake's skull called a "head-bolt."

"This 'head-bolt' is measuring the amount of pressure the inner-cranial swelling is exerting on his brain. Jake has a 'closed-head' trauma." John tried to sound cheerful and hopeful as he spoke in earshot of Jake...later he explained that they say when people are in a coma, they can hear you. I think I said to Jake that he was going to be ok...and we would be right around the corner in the waiting room if he needed us.

I tried to understand what all I was being told. Then our visiting time was up. We didn't want to leave. We were rounded up and herded back to our chairs and sat like robots for fear of leaning on the other and both of us crumbling to pieces.

"Why can't they stop his arms?" I wanted to know.

"They told me he would probably stop on his own. There is nothing they can do. His brain is hurt."

"I don't like it."

"I don't like it either. Nobody likes any of this."

"So what are their plans?"

"I guess it's a waiting game. If he begins to wake up, they will probably put him in a medically induced coma is the way I understood it. I think they already have given him the medicine but I am not sure. They don't need him waking up and beginning to get out of control. The danger is a stroke if the brain keeps swelling."

(We spoke monotone...and when we spoke at all, it was without emotion, in as few words as it took to be understood.)

The visits were repeated around the clock when they would let us in the ICU...sometimes they couldn't let us go in due to some procedure or crisis with Jake. When they did let us go in, we always said encouraging things, like ..."Jake, you really are doing a fine job working so hard to get better, we know it's tough. Keep up the fight even though it may get worse. Try to relax and concentrate on getting well."

We saw the numbers for the "head-bolt" drop lower as we talked to him....amazingly, the numbers would be in the 60's and 80's on some visits when we walked in and as we talked, the numbers lowered to 30 and 25. I think he felt relaxed and secure when we were there. He had to be scared to the depths of his soul and we were his comforters....his Mom and his Dad.

We were told the highest number on an un-injured person is around 15 and that is when we are boiling mad!

So you see how critical his pressure was and how close he was to having a stroke; even worse, to die if the extreme pressure ruptured the membrane at the top of the vertebral column and dumped his brain-matter into his spine. Death would be instant. We felt as if we were sitting on a keg of dynamite wondering when it might explode.

Knowing the danger he was in, we diligently coached him: "Hey, son. It's Mom and Dad! We know you are hurting but we know you can do this...God is helping you hang on so we feel good about you. God loves you, Jake. We are praying for you to get better so we can all go home. Son, we don't like to see you hurt like this but it is a bad hurt and will take time to heal up. You are so loved. Everyone is saying prayers for you."

We reported to him about the activities of each of his brothers and sisters and his friends so he wouldn't feel out of the loop. We gave him reports of his best friend who had come out of coma and was moved to another floor. We continuously told him we were so proud of him for trying so hard...all the kinds of positive message conversations we could muster and with a tone of reassurance to our voices to keep his spirits up to hang on….not give up….not die….not leave us.

After 72 straight hours or about 3 or 4 days, one of his arms slowed down and then quit the inhuman task of lifting the imaginary bar-bells. Just one arm was working away at the gruesome gesture…the "posturing" and I had hope again that he could avoid a heart attack or stroke.

Finally, both arms were still. My heart was so hurt for him. I wanted to be the one lying in that bed in his place. I didn't want him to be barely clinging to life…to an uncertain future. I wanted that fate to be mine not his.

The neurosurgeon stopped us in the hallway a few days into the ordeal. My brother, Jackson, had come to the hospital and was standing with us in the hall when the doctor said we needed to let Jake go. He said Jake was going to be a vegetable. It would be a miracle if he returned to his pre-wreck self. We stood dumbfounded.

I popped off, "No! Don't you dare let Jake die. Keep doing everything you can to keep him alive. Dr. Jesus is on this case, too. You just do everything you can for him...and when you can't do anything more then I'll take my vegetable home and give him Miracle-Gro."

The doctor never offered to unplug him again.

About this doctor: He was probably the second best neurosurgeon in the nation; the other one being in Boston. In many ways, we were lucky people to have a doctor of his caliber. I just wish he had been receptive to me and my ideas to help save my son – or, to have been kind enough to have taken time to explain why my thoughts were impractical.

My job was hauling chemicals in a tank trailer. I knew the principles of pressurizing and of relieving pressure on the product I hauled. Some things anatomical are just a matter of plumbing and basic physics in my opinion...and to a certain extent, that is the truth. I tried to consult with him about how I used reduction valves, levers and gauges to control the speed of relieving pressure in a pressurized tanker. The underlying principle would be the same...equalize the pressure inside his skull to that on the outside...I asked the doctor if he could prevent the pressure from continuing to build in his skull.

His answer touted the success rate of a drug called Mannitol for drawing fluid off the brain thus controlling inner-cranial pressure. It was a powerful osmotic diuretic.

I had one shot and I knew it...I tried to sound professional as I cautiously asked how about physically instead of chemically-- equalizing the inner-cranial pressure and then as soon as the pressure was under control, surgically take away a portion of his skull and replace it when the swelling had gone down.

This great doctor, as politely as I had been, explained that upon cutting into the skull, the grey matter was under pressure and would explode and just flow everywhere....and he announced that Jake would instantly be dead at that point.

He seemed to have no clue of what I was suggesting. So, I went on to ask if he could consider easing the pressure off with a reduction type method of inserting small drainage tubes and graduate up to larger and larger until enough fluid drained and the pressure was where it was safe to make an incision. I attempted to explain how, in my work, I was utilizing a system such as what I was describing on a 6500 gallon tanker with the contents under 120 psi of pressure....I tried to explain how regulating this pressure with valves and levers and gauges and hoses of various sizes so that the contents would not blast the product uncontrolled out of the tanker was crucial to safe delivery of product coming out of the pressurized tank.

Man, was I boring him. I could see it in his eyes, I had lost him....he was not listening to me. I was dismissed.

I felt abandoned. At that moment, I wished I had stayed in Pre-Med at Fresno State College, gone to medical school and had the title of M.D. after my name. Maybe then I would have had enough knowledge of the physiology of the brain to have never brought up any hare-brained solutions.

Looking back, I recall a touch of arrogance on his part. The truth is that I could have been a medical professional just like him ...and he may not have listened even then. I like to think that if I had been another doctor, he would have at least said: that won't work and you know it.

Recently, I had a surgeon friend explain to me that the severely bruised brain tissue was continually manufacturing more "product" unlike the static load I had in a tanker. When I took on 6500 gallons of a chemical, the load was never going to make more of itself/increase. The brain, as living tissue, reacts in ways that I didn't understand...especially a bruised brain. It "floats" in cerebrospinal fluid, the same stuff that bathes the spinal cord.

The brain is quite well supported inside the head and although it is floating in this bath of CSF (Cerebrospinal Fluid), actually, there are various supporting structures which help to hold the brain in one position. There is a piece of tissue called the falx cerebri which inside your skull holds your brain and stops it from going side to side or bouncing like a gelatinous ball off all the interior sides of the skull.

At the back of the head there is also a structure called the tentorium cerebelli which is a horizontal piece of tissue which holds the brain vertically and there are also the main meninges which go around the brain and they provide a degree of support as well.

When Jake's skull took that extremely tremendous hit, his brain did bounce against the other side and back... and very possibly back again. Many of the areas of support to his brain were seriously damaged. Capillaries were seeping blood and fluids as the structures they supplied were torn and ripped from their stations. These "bleeds" were increasing pressure as they vied for space inside his head.

My friend went on to explain that a doctor never knows for sure if you do cut into the skull and remove a section, whether or not the injured brain will grotesquely expand out from the opening and ever shrink back again. You cannot be guaranteed that it won't continue to enlarge and be a larger problem....so it is best that a surgeon learns some important concepts early in his career. One big lesson is that as much as he might want to do something, it is best to "sit on his hands" as my ex-flight surgeon friend so aptly put it.

I can imagine a crisis-oriented surgeon would want to do something for his suffering patient, even if it is wrong....and as my friend pointed out, some doctors learn the hard way that the wrong move can sometimes not be corrected. It is best to "sit on your hands" if there is any doubt in the picture.

The Waiting

Neither John nor I ever left that ICU Waiting Room area for any reason, 28 solid days and nights....we never left that floor (the 5th?) to go down to the cafeteria nor outside for a breath of fresh air. Our only exercise was the walk to the ICU and back to our chairs. We were not hungry but people brought food anyway. I guess we ate. I don't remember. My cousin, Marion, brought a home-cooked meal to us. I know she went to a lot of trouble but I don't remember what it was or how it tasted.

I do recall a church ministry that brought a basket of tuna fish sandwiches around daily...I always meant to write them a thank you for serving the frightened families of unfortunates such as we, and many others in that particular waiting room, were. I meant to say thanks to their group, to my cousin for her kindness shown. I wonder if it's too late?

I am a "food person" so for me not to be able to recollect a nice meal is telling you how devastated I was. We were traumatized.

I honestly believe we have suffered from undiagnosed/untreated PTSD for many years now. All of Jake's family and his family of friends were traumatized....his best friend was driving him home and that entire family was as hurt as anyone at the results of the accident. Post Traumatic

Shock Disorder. Undiagnosed and as dangerous and deadly as physical trauma if left untreated….yep, we all had ALL that.

Those of us who have survived still have a battle with PTSD.

During the time spent in the waiting room, someone found an abandoned old shower area next to where we were camped out. We slept stretched out on the barely padded, green cushioned chairs shoved together. The shower was used at one time in the past by the doctors. It still worked…we cleaned it up and used it. I think family members brought us fresh clothes. Surely they did…all I remember is the fact that we didn't want to leave our 24/7 posts.

We dared not be waiting if Jake woke up and called for us…..we also did not address it, even to ourselves, but if they came to tell us he was dying, we didn't want him to die alone…we would be by his side….we were both there when he was born….it would only be right.

A friend came to see us and in the course of conversation, all the color went out of my husband's face the moment she reached over and patted him on the knee and said, "John, I am so sorry. I am so sorry."

When she left, he told me of a dream he had about 6 months ago in May. He remembered it when she touched his knee. In the dream, this very woman was sitting across from him on a green naugahyde couch and, in the dream, she had reached out and patted him on his knee as she said, "John, I am so sorry."

He told me that this must have been a father's premonition.

On November 17th, my Daddy's birthday, 12 days after the wreck…he got a nice present. Jake was weaned off the breathing machine and breathing on his own!

Hallelujah! Praise the Lord! Jake could breathe again! We all felt thankful and now had more hope for more progress. We gave praises to God and prayed more fervently than before for God to continue to grant healing grace. It definitely seemed a good sign that, God willing, Jake would continue to improve. We took it as that. We needed hope so we could continue to give hope to Jake….and to our children and Jake's friends.

For some reason, the good doctor decided enough Mannitol had been administered and took him off the drug. This Mannitol which, by his own admission, was his only known way to control the inner-cranial pressure was discontinued....and the next 24 hours brought unbearable news; Jake had suffered four, severe, deep mid-brain strokes.

I wanted to put my hands around somebody's throat. I had to will myself to contain my anger. I physically felt hope drain out of me. The road to recovery just got more difficult.

The damage was done and irreversible...and, if I "acted up" there was a chance I would be removed from the premises. (They had already told my husband to send the upset children and their friends home or we all could leave.)

How do people make it through real tragedies without faith in a living, loving God? I don't think they do. I have had a lot of time to think on this. In my opinion: suicides and divorces, murders and other negative actions and consequences are due many times to a person not being able to cope because of lack of real faith in God. They have no hope. They have no depth of purpose nor direction to go in. They have become inwardly focused and are left with demons of their own making. They neither receive love nor have love to give. They easily turn to alcohol and drugs to dull their pain.

Those people either never knew God in their lives or for some reason (trauma) had rejected the concept of God as a loving Father in Heaven who would "let" bad things happen. They refuse to believe they cannot go on without His love. They refuse to believe He is a God of unconditional love and forgives them when they will not forgive themselves. Their lives become like a battery trying to recharge itself; it cannot sustain itself...and, at some point, the battery completely ceases to provide power. The devil loves a weakened mind. He moves in for the kill.

On the 28th day, we got word that Jake was stable enough to be transferred to Doctor's

Hospital a few miles away. We were told about the Ronald McDonald House because at the next hospital, families were expected to come to the patients' small rooms to visit and then leave; not allowed to hang out in a waiting room as we did at LSU-Med. We were not going to be allowed to hover as we were doing. A lady talked to me about the harsh reality that one of us needed to return to our job.

I had forgotten there was another thing to do in this world and I wanted nothing more but be as close to Jake as was allowed...to talk to our other children on the phone and assure them that all the things humanly possible were being done to help their brother.

[This was a total lie to my way of thinking but I became very convincing in the telling of it. I kept my true opinion and my thoughts to myself. (Secretly, I had begun to despise the medical community, one neurosurgeon in particular, for not listening to me when I begged them to open his skull and relieve the pressure that eventually caused 4 deep mid-brain strokes.) If only I had been informed all those years ago by the doctor, my thoughts would not have been nibbled on by doubts that Jake was in good hands. I felt disappointment and anger and rage but gave to my children and friends only the positives that we were told.]

Go back to work? Who, me? How could I feel good about abandoning my vigil?   I couldn't. The last thing I wanted to do was go back to my job as a trucker. In a way, I owed it to Jake to get back on the road. He was the one who had found that truck for me!

In his junior year in high school, he worked weekends at an oil change business and knew firsthand the good care given to this truck by its previous owner.

Jake made a deal with me that he would go to UTI in Houston to earn his credentials as a diesel engine mechanic when he graduated from high school. We would have our own trucking company; comprised of me and a few others driving our trucks and he would be our main shop mechanic.

"We will be uptown, Mama!"

So, with that on my mind, I spoke to my comatose son…."Hey, Jake…it's Mama. I gotta make a run to Laredo in our truck. 610 miles from Magnolia, AR where I pick up. Oughta pay good. I know you don't want me to lose our truck so I gotta make this run…Daddy will be here for you. Well…..just know I will be thinking of you and see you as soon as I get back to town."

That was the longest 610 miles I have ever driven…..I must have stopped at every rest area to try to find a phone and call the nurse's station. For some reason, I didn't have a cell phone back then and not many of the rest areas had working phones. I had not shed a tear since the night of the wreck…and those were of happiness at the wedding ceremony….now, water was welling up and overflowing as I tried to see the road ahead. My throat was constricted. I felt as if I had the band of an oil-filter wrench tightening around my neck.

The tight band couldn't be removed…later I had chest pains….people die of broken hearts..... stress was a constant.... people die of stress.

I had to "Let go and let God" or park the truck.

Christmas was around the corner....we got a cheery Santa's hat for Jake. He looked more like himself but he still had not opened his pretty blue eyes. He was able to squeeze your hand weakly. Little Tyler was the only family member with a big happy smile since he was way too young to understand any of this.

We will always be thankful for his brand of sunshine consistently given to us on all the dark days. (All he did was love and expect to be loved in return. He would smile and we had to smile back! Tyler was the best Rx we could have been prescribed. He kept us all going with his true innocence which we didn't want to ever see taken away.)

Jake was still unresponsive. It was almost Father's Day.

My good friend, Dr. Joe Mitchell Smith, had opened a rehab hospital. He got hold of me. He told me that he would like to try to work with Jake. He would handle having him transferred to Ruston.

I jumped at the chance. John was now driving back and forth to Shreveport daily; the family was under stress as never before.

Our other children were feeling completely neglected by us as well as devastated over their brother....Elisabeth was having guilt feelings that if she had not had her wedding then Jake would not have been hurt. (All her fault...) What a blessing being at the new rehab hospital in Ruston would be. So convenient for the family...and, who knows, with friends and family easily able to drop by to see him, he just might come out of the coma. You never knew what might "bring him around" and we desperately wanted him back to his "pre-wreck self" and for our lives to get back on a normal schedule that we could handle.

You cannot make it through without your faith in God.

In the telling of what happened to our family as we dealt with Traumatic Brain Injury, I am realizing what a destructive role TBI played in our family and how it has lead up to so many other regrettable and completely unnecessary situations that have given us sleepless nights in fear for the safety of one child or another, tested our patience, our love for each other and our confidence in ourselves to make a decision that is best for all concerned.

You are never prepared. You don't raise your family and ever once catch yourself saying: Now children, I want you to listen up: here is what we do when one of you gets brain-injured.

We will invest in a special wheelchair; we will build ramps to wheel you in the house. We will buy a special van with a lift and we will buy a hospital bed and a sling to get you in and out of the tub and have all sorts of therapy lined up for you to regain use of your body in case you come out of your coma. Your brothers and sisters will take you in your wheelchair to ballgames and to parties as you continue to heal...

No, you won't say those things to prepare your family because you have no clue about what happens. It is an entirely different world. It can be compared to planning to go live in Germany. You spend years in making your preparations. You are learning the German language and after years of study, you become proficient in speaking German. You get on a plane for your flight over and when you land, you discover that somehow you end up on Mars and there's not enough fuel to return. That's crazy, you say? Well, that's how crazy it is.

No, you cannot ever prepare yourself or your family for TBI. You don't know to do that. Nobody plans to have a family member with TBI. The price you pay to walk that ground is high and is never what you expect. Your losses will far outweigh your gains but it is possible to make it through by the decisions you make if you allow God to play a major role in helping you as a parent, spouse or child of a person with TBI.

I am not kidding about having enough faith to accept whatever God puts in your life. I am a terrible Christian who is not always in the church house every Sunday morning but running up and down the nations' highways. My husband is there every time the doors are open.

If I can be as sinful and full of faults as I am, and the likes of me is trying to tell you that God in our lives is the only answer, you need, there must be something to it. He is the only one who can make the difference we are looking for...the Bible is the living word of the Lord and to prove that truth to yourself...pick it up when you are trouble and see that He speaks to you from that book as appropriately as can be done. Try it.

He is the only one who truly loves us unconditionally.

The role that TBI played in our family has many times tested our ability to hang on to our sanity and composure until we were down to the last ounce of strength; miraculously we have somehow been left with just enough good judgment to take that little bit of strength and give our troubles up to God. We find we are okay when we have finally quit being stubborn and have let Him take on the weight of our hopelessness and helplessness; and, then He shows us that it is all good and so much better than when we were trying to be strong and go it alone.

I do hope the story of Jake's tragedy is found in time to be helpful to those who have to endure dark hours of facing the unknown. Maybe just one little thing I may say in telling what happened to my child and how it has all but torn our family apart will help another family circumvent the potholes of this lonesome highway.

We have tried to cling together through the storms of life during and after Traumatic Brain Injury. We, the McCann Family, are still making our way. It is still not an easy path. You never know for certain what is around the next bend in the road.

At the time the crisis happens, you may be like me and try to strike a deal with God. You may find yourself alone one night as I did down in Marfa, Tx. I shut my engine off and listened to the silence. I got out wondering if it was rattlesnake season...and climbed up on my trailer so as not to be bothered. I have never been where it was so quiet; it was in one moment as a cathedral and yet as a tomb.

I could hear the blood rushing in my ears before every beat of my heart.

No city lights to pollute the view of all the stars above. With my chest aching from hurting over Jake, I stood there on top of my flatbed trailer in the desert surroundings and gazed up into the canopy of the black sky with all the pinpricks of stars. I had never seen so many little stars up there. It brings home how small and insignificant we are......I started out talking prayerfully to God in His Heaven....told him how strikingly beautiful this world was that He prepared for us....then I became irrationally angry and more and more angry as I recounted things to do with Jake's situation...and the fact that none of us could enjoy anything because Jake had lost the ability to enjoy anything.

Next thing I knew, I had "lost it" and screamed with terrible might into the darkness...I did not know a human could be as loud as I was. I have never heard anyone drag out the length of our Creator's name as I did that night. I feel shame in recounting it but I want to share it in case another sinner has a melt-down over their child whose brain is all but destroyed. I want that other bereft sinner like me to know God can handle getting yelled at...it is not a nice thing to do to the one who loves us as much as He does.

I bellowed up to the stars: "God! I know you are there. I know you hear me. What are you gonna do for Jake? Are you listening? I'm gonna offer this one more time, God, and you gotta do it. You take ME in his place. I don't care if you cast me straight into hell...You hear me, Lord! Me, damn it! (Tears here...and I fall to my knees....) Not my child. Not my Jake...No! No! Nooooooo! You can't have him. He hasn't even lived his life. I'm begging you. Lord...just get me...get me now...get it over with...I am ready to go. Call off that angel of death or whatever you have going after Jake...send death to me now. I mean it."

I howled and carried on out there like something loosed from the bowels of hell itself. I woke up before dawn because I was cold.

I felt badly about acting out like that...if a rattler had bitten me, I would have figured I deserved it. I told God I meant every word of it but I was sorry I said it and I hoped He could forgive me.

Believe me, and I am sure you do, you honestly don't want to live if there is any way your child can be spared by your own act of dying.

I will go so far as to tell you that I went about it all wrong.... the only prayer I should have prayed over and over was,

"Not my will, but yours, Lord."

(I recommend this prayer as the most wise prayer when searching for the workable answer to your troubles. He has a plan; it will prevail, sooner or later.)

Gabriel put it in terms we could identify with….he said, "Jake's life is a phone call and somebody pushed the hold button; it is still waiting to be answered."

I worried how this son would take the ordeal…Jake was as near to being his twin as two brothers could be. When Gabriel was born, my Daddy announced, "Jake's twin is here…just two years late!"

It became obvious over the next years and is now: Gabe put his own life on hold and to this day has not resumed it as he needs to…Unresolved grief? PTSD? Maybe both.

Whatever it is, it is a terrible, heartfelt, soul-deep pain to deal with...and he doesn't handle it well at all....we see the same signs of unresolved grief in his sister and his big brother...and ourselves. We are "some kind of messed up"...by the Grace of a loving Heavenly Father, we are all forgiven and even though, we backslide sometimes, we are okay....not immune to mistakes and heartaches and pain but we are okay because God is in our lives and we want Him here.

We have been told by some well-meaning friends that we need to find "closure"....and, try as we may, we can't do it. I conclude that you don't find closure, not ever, not really...I think it is just an illusion to believe you have found closure. To me, "closure" is just a word tossed around when people are tired of feeling grief or tired of hearing you talk about your feeling of loss.

The Therapist

We were looking for ways to cope. It felt as if we had gotten up one morning and war had been declared on our family. We had one man down and the rest of us were the "walking wounded." Someone suggested family counseling. The rehab hospital had a psychologist on staff.

I need to make the remark for the record that we were given more respect and concern and caring at that hospital than any facility could have offered our family. Jake had the most up-to-date treatment available and a doctor and his staff who truly cared about Jake.

Every Tuesday evening, John and I, Daddy and his wife, Elisabeth and her new husband, Gabriel and even little Tyler...the exception was our oldest boy who was working out of state. We were to assemble as a group in the cafeteria at the rehab hospital. After several sessions, that left us as dazed as we were when we arrived, I asked the therapist to explain why it was when we asked questions, he countered us with a question of his own, never one time offering us even a tidbit of information to help us heal?

I sincerely wanted answers to my questions. I believed the others wanted answers to their questions and told him so. We had to get help and soon! Our relationships were falling apart and we were all losing sleep and trying to make sense of "sense-less" which cannot be done.

"So, how can you help us?"

His answer stunned me.

"Oh ...let me explain. You may not know it but I am in the process of writing a thesis for my doctorate. It is on 'The Effects of Traumatic Brain Injury Patients on Their Family Members.'"

Immediately, the hope I had allowed to rebuild drained right out of my being as it had done when Jake had the four strokes in one night.

I felt demoted. I no longer held the status of the mother of a son who had been tragically, terribly hurt. I now held the status of the mother guinea pig in a lab setting.

We were a completely and absolutely devastated family under the microscope. We were under observation in a Petri dish of some barely fathomable fashion where we floated around on the surface as life-forms. Various needles poked and jabbed at us; we recoiled with the pain of these needles which took the form of daily disappointments in the lack of response by Jake to the wonderful care and treatment he was being given. Our son's critically injured body and brain just would not co-operate and heal but developed more complications and maladies which were not compatible with normal life.

At the time, all of this horror was too new for us to find a handle to grasp for support; consequently, we found ourselves hit gut-level and knocked to our knees each time a malady cropped up….we did not know so much could go so wrong. Jake was a good son…he did not deserve to suffer….and we all suffered right along with him.

I think he knew and was saddened to know he was the reason for so much pain and sorrow. He was the one we had always called the "Peace-maker" of the family…the one who could resolve conflicts and hurts…now he was hurt and so were we….and, we still hurt.

With no understanding of Traumatic Brain Injury which the professionals called TBI for short, we had no real hope and no idea where to go to change the situation. There were no books to read. No experts to consult. We knew of another family in town who also had a child with TBI and they explained they had no more answers than we had. TBI seems to be different with every patient.

We were as injured as if we had been in the wreck with Jake...we were in need of help and our world was never far from his hospital bed. It didn't matter if we were in line at the grocery store or driving down the highway, we were really right at that bedside where Jake lay in coma. We were all damaged beyond repair. I believe we were as close to a diagnosis of Post Traumatic Stress Disorder as a person can be.

My opinion in 2013 is that we each needed treatment for PTSD in 1995. I believe some of the heart-rending and unfortunate personal experiences and additional tragedies our family has experienced in the years after Jake was hurt could have been avoided. We had no help with our mental health from the medical community. A dark cloud hung overhead in each of our lives. The joy of a sun-kissed morning, the music of chirping birds and the lush beauty of nature surrounding us --was simply now a sad reminder that Jake could not see all this anymore. No bright sunshine, no colorful rainbows, no breath-taking sunrises and sunsets for Jake in coma; for that reason, we had no pleasure either...if he couldn't share in it, we didn't even want it.

Hunting and fishing and vacations were all put on a back-burner for a better time. (A better time never came.) If we saw young couples, about his age, strolling together, it was another reminder that Jake more than likely will never live a normal life. He will never be able to marry the girl of his dreams and have his own family.

Our own dreams for Jake were fading fast as we realized how seriously he was injured. The letter we got from Doctor's Hospital to admit him to the North Louisiana Rehabilitation Hospital said he was "permanently and completely disabled physically and mentally...would be confined to a nursing facility all the days of his life."

A nursing home? Our child? No...that's for old people! Your children are supposed to put you in one of those places. This is all backwards! We needed help!!

What we got was a therapist who (to his credit) was honest enough to admit his true motive was to obtain personal achievement. If we got helped in the process, then so be it. No...I would not have this!

I thought it out. Yes, it would be all the better for the ambitious psychologist if we flunked the part about our question being answered with another question from him…who did he think he was? Socrates?

If this line of thinking, this type of therapy, were allowed to continue then our trauma and distress would open up avenues for his study while we continued to flounder and nurse our heartbreak. How sad.

(I had one semester in college of psychology….I remember that the Socratic method was used to get a person to answer his own questions by asking him a series of questions. Well, hell's bells! No way is a devastated family, such as we were at that time, going to be able to answer their own questions. The wounds were just too fresh.)

We had never walked that ground before. We were lost, afraid and unhappy and had no idea how to change our situation.

It would have been better if the therapist had told us up front: Hey, I feel for you folks but I have absolutely no answers. It is regrettably all up to you to figure out your dilemma. On the other hand, if you want to take part in my experiment...

We desperately wanted and needed help so we could take stock of where we were and find out how to remain strong for each other and for Jake at that time --and also when he came out of the deep coma.

Moments after his admission of the doctoral work, I remember becoming coherent enough to ask him if he had ever seen anyone dealing with this kind of thing before. He had no answer; all that struck me was that he had no words of assurance for me or any of us in our grief-state.

The little fire of hope inside my heart was immediately snuffed out. The realization that this man could not help my family was crushing. Actuality: we were on our own and had been. We had no one directing us to mental health again....no one with answers to guide us.

My husband, my father and his wife agreed that we advise the family not to go back to the sessions....continue to deal with it best we could by leaning on the Lord and each other as well as supportive friends. We probably prayed more in the first 6 months than we had in all of life to that point.

At this writing in 2013, I don't instantly recall the events in any sequence, but many thoughts are surfacing now. I am overdue in writing the story of what happened so many years ago. I imagine a number of people could have been helped by hearing Jake's story but I just couldn't do this until now.

On a personal level, in the present telling of what happened to our family as we dealt with Traumatic Brain Injury, I can understand what has lead up to other regrettable situations that have tested our patience, our love for each other, our confidence in ourselves, even tested our ability to hang on to the last ounce of strength in our soul. (This strength has to be adequate for the person to have enough good judgment left to give it all up to God for survival.)

I do hope the story of Jake 's tragedy is found by someone who will be helped by knowing what happened to my child and how it all but tore our family apart as we have tried to cling together through the storms of life during and after Traumatic Brain Injury.

We held to the idea that this is God's world and His plan….not our world and not our plan. We finally adapted our lives to the knowledge that although we didn't like what had happened to Jake; nor understand why it happened; we had to do but one thing. We had to accept it.

It is not what happens in life that matters but the way what happens is handled. God has become our main therapist.

Jake's life affected so many more than just his family.

Good things can sometimes come of bad things. In the months after his death, we were humbled by so many stories of what he meant in the lives of others.

One account that will always stick with me is a story we learned from the mother of a little boy. The school bus would drop her son off at the nursing home where he would have to stay until her shift as a nurse was over. Jake's room was directly across from the nurse's station.

The curious little boy could not help but notice a young man on a bed completely enclosed with mesh...much like you see as a safety net on a trampoline. (Jake could move his legs enough to turn his body and tumble out of his bed. Sadly, one occasion, when a nursing assistant forgot to zip the enclosure after his late night meds were administered through his stomach-tube, we got a call that he was in the ambulance headed to the ER. Jake had crashed to the floor and lacerated his head on the bedside table.)

(My Daddy would go out to the nursing home and sit with Jake to give John a break or let him go get a hamburger and check on the other children.) One day, my Daddy had been visiting with this articulate youngster; and, thinking that he was an older child than he actually was, got out the photo album.

He never would have showed a ten year old any of those pictures of the wrecked vehicle with Jake's blood and the glass everywhere. The boy was entranced as he looked them over. You can imagine the impact this had on him of seeing the wrecked truck and then looking over at Jake in a semi-comatose state in the odd bed.

My father told this child how drinking and driving don't mix. He told the little boy that he hoped his family would never have to experience anything like what Jake's family was going through.

He explained it was due to Jake's bad choice of letting a friend who had been drinking drive him home. Jake's decision got him hurt bad. Jake's decision caused his best friend who was driving and his best friend's family and all who loved him the kind of pain that you cannot describe in words.

After Jake died, the nurse wrote a letter that her son had gone home that very evening and told her husband all about Jake and the pictures of the wrecked truck and how he felt so sad for Jake's grandfather. Over time, her husband started coming to church with them and was able to quit his drinking and their family was happier than ever before.

If Jake's short life on earth did no more than influence just one individual, it was worth our son having lived and suffered and died.

Upon his death, we offered to donate his organs if that would help someone but they said he had been through too much and been given too many medications which rendered his organs useless.

When we cleaned out his room at the nursing home, all of his earthly belongings fit in only two cardboard boxes! My first thought was how terribly sad for all you own to fit into a couple of boxes. Then it came home to me, an accumulation of material things you leave behind are not what count in this life. I don't think Jesus even owned a pillow for his head.

Jake had been to a Jay Strack Campus Crusade for Christ at LA TECH University. It was on a night in May when he gave his heart to Jesus. He was injured in November. We feel good about his spiritual life.

In 2nd Samuel, verse 12: King David said when his son died, He may not can come to me but I can go to him. David trusted in the Lord for his own salvation and believed he would go to Heaven and be able to see his son again.

We have assurance we will see our son again.

EPILOGUE

The time was November 5th, 1995 when our middle son was involved in a serious wreck that ended his life as we knew it and left him trapped in a virtually useless body for 5 years, 5 months, 22 days, 9 hours and 8 minutes. He died on April 29, 2000; just 24 days short of turning 24.

We opened a trucking business and hired more drivers to help me with the freight hauling.

I thought about Jake making plans for the future and how he intended to be our main mechanic.

He said, "We will be "Uptown, Mama!"

So, in his honor, we named the business

UPTOWN TRUCKING COMPANY.

JAMES JACOB MCCANN

Born May 22nd 1976 in Ruston, LA to Marion Biggs McCann and John Otis McCann He died on April 29th 2000 from injuries sustained on November 5th, 1995. He leaves behind his sisters, Johnette, Jessica and Elisabeth. His brothers, John Carroll and Gabriel McCann and many cousins and nephews and nieces along with his many friends, employers and teachers.

We know beyond the shadow of any doubt that God loves each of us beyond our comprehension. He is with us in the worst of times.

He will see each of us through to the end of our life on His earth.

It was a privilege to have been gifted with a son whose life was a positive influence even as he bravely lay upon the worst bed of affliction imaginable. When we finally learn that there is truly a purpose to everything under Heaven, inclusive of the most painful life-events, we will find comfort in that knowledge.

We learned that a purpose can be unknown and completely invisible to mortal man and it is okay and worthy of trust that all will turn out fine.

Faith is the difference between the Heaven-bound and the Hell-bent.

At this writing, it is going on 18 years since the wreck and as for our therapist: I learned he was a good man who loved the Lord but for some reason in dealing with us, he left God out of the equation. In so doing, he was inadequate for my family's needs.

Regrettably, I have come to know firsthand and much in-depth all about the topic our therapist was researching.

"The Effects of TBI on the Patient's Family Members"

I can write that thesis for him!

Our Second Encounter with TBI

Our family went through quite a fright last year. August 6th 2012, Tyler's Sergeant called. I saw the look on John's face as he repeated the officer's rank and name and started walking away from Stormy and me. I heard John ask what time it took place. That is when I moved to take her in the house and see if we could find a cartoon on TV. Settling her on the sofa, I hurried back outside in time to hear John say he appreciated being alerted of Tyler's injuries by phone and that he felt we were among the fortunate not to have soldiers in uniform getting out of a car in our driveway bringing worse news.

Our 19 year old Tyler was injured in Afghanistan about 4 hours prior to the phone call. (Yes, this is the same little Mr. Sunshine. He is all grown up now! He had proven himself a soldier in the summer of 2011 and gone over to fight the Taliban. He was a crack-shot sniper and soon became an expert mortar gunner.)

Briefly, I will tell you what happened. He was coming back with his unit in one of those relatively safe Stryker vehicles with the "V" shaped hull to deflect explosive devices. His was the 5th vehicle in the convoy and they are told they ran over two 90-pound bombs...they were also told that the "V" hull of their Stryker vehicle became shaped like the letter "C" from the impact of these Taliban IED's planted in the roadway. (IED stands for Improvised Explosive Device.)

Tyler told us they were returning from a mission over a stretch of road the National Guard had recently been working on. They felt fairly safe! In fact, they were napping.

His Stryker commander was driving and got hurt the very worst; was flown to Germany to have pins put in his shattered legs. Tyler was next in degree of injury...and their medic was also hurt so medics from the other vehicles came to assist all the injured troops.

Tyler had his helmet on and the impact turned on the head-cam so if he ever wants to relive those moments, its on video. He reports trying to grab a rifle to set up a defense not realizing he had a fractured shoulder, nerve damage to one hand and his ankles messed up. They were in hill country and had jeeps to come get them moved out. The medics gave 'em morphine for the pain of transport over the terrain to the areas where Medivac choppers would be landing, so he can't remember much after that except that they started cutting off his uniform and it was the only one he had left in good shape.

It was three days before he was able to call us from the Warrior Recovery Unit at Kandahar Air Field and he explained that as soon as they could get him stabilized, he would be headed to Landstul Regional Medical Center in Germany for surgery and rehab. This is the largest American hospital outside the United States.

Aside from other injuries sustained in the blast from IED's, he was diagnosed with mild-TBI. (In our family, we don't consider TBI and the word "mild" to go together. This news hurt us to the quick as a floodgate opened and memories came rushing back.)

You can imagine the anxiety it caused us to hear that term again and wonder what the outcome would be this time around. (After 5 months in re-hab, we think he is going to be fine.)

So you see, I have another reason to get Jake's story out there. I want to offer encouragement to families facing life with TBI. I am hearing more about TBI than ever before due to war injuries. The sheer number of our wounded warriors and disabled veterans is regrettably on the rise.

Back then, 1995, I searched for information to inform us but found none. I asked my Daddy to go find me any book or pamphlet that had head trauma in its title and bring it to the waiting room. I needed answers. I needed to understand what we were dealing with. He came up with a few...and even one to do with magnetic resonance imaging. I scanned and sifted through all he found. Some were text book quality but written in generalities. He found nothing describing what had happened, what was happening and what could happen to our patient.

Perhaps back then, not only was there not much on TBI but the information I needed and was searching for is so personal--is so sad for a person to recount, so hard to write that I can understand now why it was not in abundance.

I don't recall using the Internet. (Did we have it in 1995?) There is more information than you may want out there now. Then there are folks such as myself wanting to lend support by recounting and writing their experience with a loved one's TBI.

The work being done with head trauma patients these days is more than adequate and the research is on-going. Physical and mental therapist are light years ahead of what was available for Jake. There are special appliances and apparatus and programs to take advantage of and more to come. Your experience will be tolerable but not one of choice. I do hope this act of recording our ordeal with Jake may give you some enlightenment or help someone you know. It stands to reason that it may help me more than anyone. They say writing is therapeutic.

Never leave God out of the equation.

I am not trying to cheer you up. I am here to help you be braced for whatever comes your way with your patient. It has been a terrible time for us over all the years. Even now, when we see a reminder of Jake, we grieve our loss of him. If a well-meaning person finds photos with him in it and sends them to us, it is a stab in the heart to see Jake at a time in our family when the circle was unbroken.

You would not wish Traumatic Brain Injury on your worst enemy's child.

END

www.ingramcontent.com/pod-product-compliance
Lightning Source LLC
Chambersburg PA
CBHW051329170526
45166CB00002B/736